I0423356

Fat Is Your Friend

Why Eating The Right Fats Are Key For Healthy Weight Loss and Feeling Great

JJ Miller

© 2016

Disclaimer

All rights reserved. No part of this publication may be reproduced, distributed, or transmitted in any form or by any means, including photocopying, recording, or other electronic or mechanical methods, without the prior written permission of the publisher, except in the case of brief quotations embodied in critical reviews and certain other noncommercial uses permitted by copyright law.

This book is not intended as a substitute for the medical advice of physicians. The reader should regularly consult a physician in matters relating to his/her health and particularly with respect to any symptoms that may require diagnosis or medical attention.

Fat Is Your Friend:

Why Eating The Right Fats Are Key For Healthy Weight Loss And Feeling Great

Introduction

What is fat and why is it so important?

Fat by definition is one of the three nutrients used in the body as energy. They energy that is produced by fat is higher than protein, and carbohydrates at 9 calories per gram. When you see total fat amounts of on nutrition label this is the sum of all saturated fat, monounsaturated fats, as well as polyunsaturated fat. Fat is an extremely important component to overall health, and our bodies need a certain amount of healthy fats in order to function properly.

What most people do not know is that our brains are made up of nearly 60% fat! What this means is that without adding dietary fat to our diets our brains are not able to function optimally. Fat is also crucial for hormone balance, energy levels, as well as assisting our bodies in absorbing essential vitamins and minerals. Fat is also essential to maintain healthy hair, and skin and fat is responsible for insulating our cells to help to keep our bodies warm. (1) There are also different types of fats, and it's required to get certain fats from foods, since our bodies cannot synthesize them. These fats are called essential fatty acids and are necessary for brain health, to fight inflammation as well as for blood clotting.

Consuming fats, and specifically the healthy kinds of fats is crucial to helping our bodies function at the level that it needs to.

Our Misconception of Fat:

Over the years fat has received a bad reputation. There have been so many fad diets promoting low fat to fat free, and so many marketing companies advertising low fat snacks and poor education our there educating the public on how low fat or skim milk is the way to go if you want to stay slim and healthy. Unfortunately all of the mixed messages that are out there today about fat, are just not true, and can actually harm our health in the long run.

Since fat is needed for many functions in the body it is essential that we are consuming adequate amounts in order to nourish and care for our bodies, and feed our brains. Without dietary fat, our brains will not work as well as the should, our hormones would be out of balance, our energy levels very low, and we would see vitamin and mineral deficiencies since many vitamins require fat in order for proper absorption to occur.

There has recently been many misconceptions about fat because of what mainstream news and media is telling us. One of the biggest misconceptions of fat is that foods high in dietary fat such as eggs will raise our cholesterol levels. The recent studies on eggs have shown that they have the ability to raise HDL cholesterol, which is the healthy kind of cholesterol and the kind we want more in our diets. Eggs are loaded with vitamins, minerals, and healthy fats and should not be avoided. So whenever you hear someone say to ditch the egg yolk, and stick with the egg white know that the yolk is what holds the nutrients and what is going to fuel our bodies with what it needs.

Another misconception about fats is that dietary fats will make us fat, and that we should be eating low fat or fat free whenever it is available to us. What the fat free advertisements don't shed light on is that many low fat items are incredibly high in sugar which is actually going to lead to weight gain faster than healthy fats ever would. When it comes to fat, it's important to understand that healthy fats such as whole milk, unsweetened full fat yogurt, coconut oil, avocados, and nut butters are actually extremely healthy and when consumed in moderate portions they can actually contribute to weight loss. Throughout this book, I am going to de-bunk the fat free misconceptions and shine light on how fat can actually help to keep you lean and healthy.

Chapter 2:

Why is Fat Actually Good for you?

Why Eating Fat Doesn't make us Fat:

While this may come as a shock to many, eating fat does not actually make us fat at all! Now that we know that fat is an essential nutrient to keep our bodies going, let's discuss why exactly fats are not what is contributing to weight gain.

When you consume calories from fat, those calories are no different than the calories that you consume from carbohydrates and protein. (2) We also know that eating fat will not immediately put extra fat tissue into your body. It's similar to how protein works, just because you may consume a large amount of protein, it does not mean that the extra protein is going to immediately bulk up your muscles.

One of the major myths about fat is that fats are empty calories, and therefore will make you gain weight. This is the furthest thing from the truth, considering fat is an essential nutrient. The myth that fats are empty calories is null and void, because carbohydrates by themselves as well as protein by themselves contain zero vitamins and minerals as well. Some of the most nutrient dense foods in the world are high in fats, such as egg yolks, liver, fresh meat, dairy products, and fatty fish, and consuming these foods regularly will improve your health, not make you gain weight. Diet's high in healthy fats can help to fuel our mitochondria, provide power anti-inflammatory benefits, and can actually reduce problems with cholesterol if you are consuming the right types of fats.

Studies have been conducted on the health benefits on consuming healthy fats vs. people who restricted their fat intake and consumed a diet high in low fat foods and refined carbohydrates. The studies always prove that the people who regularly consume healthy fats have fewer health issues than those who consume a high sugar, high carbohydrate diet low in fat. Dr. Mark Hyman, saying that "Eating a diet with good quality fat and protein prevents and even reverses diabetes and pre-diabetes. And eating sugar and refined carbs cause diabesity." (3) "Diabesity", is the combination of diabetes, and obesity. So don't avoid the fat, you should actually go ahead and enjoy the fat! Ditch the low fat food label, cut back or eliminate refined carbohydrates and focus on looking at fat in a different light.

Below are some of the top healthiest fat options to include in your diet:

- Olive oil
- Nuts/Seeds

- Fatty fish

- Avocados

- Grass fed animal products

- Coconut oil

Fat and Heart Disease:

Another misconception about fat, is that fat causes heart disease. No matter how hard nutrition professionals, or those in the preventative health field try to stress the important of knowing that it is not fat that is making us sick, and overweight, it seems to always come back as a topic of conversation. The truth of the matter is that sugar is causing many more problems with our health than a healthy dose of fat will cause. Fat has been the center of attention when talking about heart disease for quite some time now. Just like how fat is thought to make us fat, we need to discuss how fat is not responsible for causing heart disease.

Out of the different types of fats, saturated fat is typically the fat that comes under fire when talking about heart disease. Chris Kresser, states that "For more than five decades we've been brainwashed to believe that saturated fat causes heart disease. It's such a deeply ingrained belief that few people even question it. It's just part of our culture now." (4) He also goes on to talk about how many people believe that a "healthy" diet consists of low fat option but that there is no evidence that supports that consuming saturated fats leads to heart disease, and that all of the studies that have stated that saturated fats are bad for our health were poorly designed, while you will not be able to find any well designed studies published in any medical journals regarding the connection between saturated fats and heart disease.

In 2010 there was a report published in the American Journal of Clinical Nutrition that stated that after a 14 year study, there was no relationship between the consumption of saturated fats and the development of heart disease or even stroke. If you still aren't convinced, think about those who follow the Mediterranean style diet that is high in things like olive oil and fatty fish. Studies have shown that women who followed a Mediterranean diet lowered their risk of heart disease by 29%. (5)

The sad truth is that over the years we have been encouraged to eat all of the wrong foods. Main stream media encourages people to consume packaged and processed foods due to the large fear many have over fat. The focus has been shifted towards consuming packaged foods as opposed to fresh, whole foods that are full of vitamins, minerals, and high quality nutrition with healthy fats to help our bodies absorb all of the nutritional value. It's important that we shed some knowledge on fat, and how fat is not what is causing the obesity epidemic, it's the foods that we have been told to eat that are full of sugar and artificial ingredients that are causing these problems.

Fat and Hormones:

In order to have harmonious hormone balance, we need to consume fat. Fats help to regulate the production of sex hormones, and without fat, teenagers may experience developmental delays which is why it is especially important to choose the whole fat versions of foods, and to consume foods that are naturally rich in dietary fat during the pre-pubescent and pubescent years. Dietary fat is also required in order to form steroid hormones that are needed in order to regulate numerous bodily processes. Fats, and especially healthy amounts of saturated fats in the diet are also especially helped for men and testosterone levels.

Without fats, our bodies would have a very difficult time in producing hormones. It's crucially important that children, and teenagers get enough healthy fat in their diet in order to produce enough hormones so they do not experience developmental delays. In adulthood dietary fats are important in order to maintain hormonal balance.

Chapter 3:

How Fats Can Make You Thinner and Healthier & Which Ones to Eat

High Fat Consumption for a Low Fat Body

By now, we know that dietary fats are essential for a healthy life, and that fats are not what is making us fat. What if I told you that consuming healthy fats can actually lead to a lower fat body? That would be some pretty exciting news, and the bottom line is that yes, fat consumption can actually lead to a leaner and healthier body.

In order to help your body shed excess fat, you will need to consume 25-30% of your total daily calories from healthy fats. Certain fats that are naturally high in healthy fats can actually help to trim your waistline. Grass-fed beef for example containers fewer calories than conventional meats, and contains higher amounts of omega-3 fatty acids which can help to prevent heart disease. Another fat fighting food is olive oil. Olive oil is a superfood that has claimed to help fight against cancer, fight inflammation and even help with weight loss. A recent study from *Obesity* was able to show that a diet high in olive oil can actually led to an increase in adiponectin levels which is the hormone that is responsible for breaking down fat in the body. The more adiponectin you have in your body the easy it will be for your body to break down excess fat. These are just a few example as to how high fat foods can actually help your body to lose weight. For more on specific foods that help keep us lean, take a look at the next section in this chapter.

Fat consumption can also lead to a leaner body because fat helps to keep you full. Fat takes more time to digest which means it sits in your digestive system a little longer than other macronutrients do. Monounsaturated fats can actually help to stabilize blood sugars, and will help keep you feeling full longer, so you won't be reaching for that sugary snack after every meal.

Fat can also help to increase muscle. Without muscle, our metabolisms would stay the same. The more muscle we have, the faster our metabolisms will be. With an increase in exercise and fats in your diet you could greatly increase your muscle mass and promote a speedy metabolism. As stated before, fat also help to absorb essential vitamins and minerals. Some of them include Vitamin A, D, E, and K other known as the fat-soluble vitamins which means that our bodies are not able to absorb these without fat. These vitamins are needed to maintain energy levels, focus and muscles which are also essential for contributing to a healthy weight. To help our bodies absorb these vitamins try adding a little olive or coconut oil to your sautéed vegetables or chopping some avocado up and tossing it in your salad.

No matter what way you look at it, fat is essential for so many body functions, and without these functions we would not be able to maintain a healthy weight or even lose weight if we needed to. Start including healthy fats into your diet and see how much easier it is to maintain that healthy weight you are striving for.

What Fats are best to Eat?

As with anything there are always going to be better choices than others, and fats are no exception. Fats have the ability to provide your body with what it needs to carry out normal body function, however there are definitely certain fats that are going to benefit your body, and certain fats that are not. Let's take a look at some of the healthiest fat choices.

1. **Olive Oil:** We have touched upon olive oil already, however olive oil is one of those fats that contains so many health benefits it's hard to even talk about them all. Olive oil has been proven to prevent and help so many diseases that this fat should be added to everyone's diet. Olive oil is loaded

with antioxidants, is high in vitamins E and K, and has been shown to be able to reduce blood pressure and high cholesterol. Olive oil is the oil of choice when you are looking for a fat to promote cardiovascular health.

2. **Avocados:** Avocados are a wonderful addition to a healthy diet, and a rich source of healthy fat. Avocados are one of the largest dietary sources of potassium, more so than bananas! They are also wonderful sources of fiber, and can also lower LDL cholesterol levels, which is the type of cholesterol we do not want in our blood. Despite the fact that avocados are very high in fat, studies have shown that those who tend to eat avocados actually lose weight and have less belly fat than those who do not enjoy this beautiful fruit. (6)

3. **Dark chocolate:** I am sure you are relieved to hear that on a healthy diet you can include a little dark chocolate in there too! Dark chocolate can be extremely healthy in moderation if you are consuming the chocolate that is at least 70% cocoa. Dark chocolate is rich in healthy fats, high in magnesium, and has also been shown to have heart health benefits. Dark chocolate can also help to improve your mood, as well as lower blood pressure.

Have you noticed a trend here? Some of the foods that are highest in fat are the same foods that hold some of the greatest heart health benefit, yet fat is still shamed and myths are still out there that fat is the culprit of heart disease.

4. **Whole Eggs:** As we have discussed previously, the whole egg is going to give you the nutritional benefit you need, not the white part of the egg. The yolk of an egg is extremely nutritionally dense and contains numerous health benefits. Eggs are high in antioxidants, and are rich in choline which is a brain nutrient that a whopping 90% of people do not get enough of! Eggs are also a weight loss friendly food, and contain protein as well as fat to keep you feeling full longer, and less likely to over eat.

5. **Fatty Fish:** I'm sure you have heard about some of the health benefits fish like salmon hold. Other fish such as trout, mackerels, sardines, and herring are also great sources of omea-3 fatty acids. They are also great sources of protein. People who eat fish are often much healthier, have a lower risk of developing heart disease as well as depression and dementia due to the high amounts of omega-3 fatty acids. If you remember, our brains are made up of nearly 60% fat. When we fuel our brains with nutrient rich fats, our chances of developing certain neurological conditions decreases as well as our risk of heart disease and obesity.

6. **Nuts:** Nut's are an excellent choice as a healthy snack or if you are looking for ways to add a little extra healthy fat into your diet. Walnuts are even a rich source of omega-3 fatty acids which is important for inflammation as well as brain health, and most nuts are a great source of magnesium. According to Authority Nutrition, those who eat nuts tend to have a lower risk of obesity, heart disease as well as Type II Diabetes.

7. **Chia Seeds:** If you are looking for a healthy fat that will help to keep your waist slim while also providing you with some pretty impressive health benefits, chia seeds are it. Chia seeds are rich in fiber, and give you a sense of satiety when consumed. These seeds are another great choice when looking for great sources of omega-3 fatty acids. Chia seeds are nearly 80% fat making them low in carbohydrates, high in fiber and a great plant-based fat which we all could use a little more of. Chia seeds can also help to lower blood pressure, and can help to fight off inflammation.

8. **Coconut Oil:** Here is another great option when looking for healthy oils. Coconut oil is a great choice is you are looking for a new healthy oil to cook with since it has a higher smoke point than olive oil. Coconut oil can also aide in weight loss and is a very powerful antibacterial and antiviral. Since coconut oil is a medium chain fatty acid, the fat is broken down differently

in the body, and this fat is able to help to suppress your appetite which can be helpful when you are watching your weight. Coconut oil can also help to boost metabolism and can actually help you to lose belly fat.

So many people have "fat phobia" when in reality certain fat's are the best foods to consume when you are trying to lose weight or stay slim.

9. **Full Fat Yogurt:** You know those low fat, or fat free yogurts you see at the grocery store? Stay away from them! These yogurts as marketed as being a "health" food when in reality they are loaded with sugar, and often times artificial ingredients. Full fat yogurt can actually be very healthy for you. When you are looking for a full fat yogurt, go for the unsweetened kind to avoid added sugars. Full fat yogurts are high in probiotics which is essential for gut health, and without proper gut health, weight loss can be difficult. Full fat yogurts can lead to improved digestion which can result in a reduced chance of developing obesity, and again heart disease.

10. **Cheese:** Here is another food that is loved by so many, and when you are looking to lose weight it is not something you have to completely give up! Just like the dark chocolate, moderation is key but cheese can actually be

very healthy for you. Cheese is high in calcium, B12, protein, and important fatty acids.

The Unhealthy Fats:

Now that we have listed to healthiest options you can make when choosing healthy fats, we need to look at the fats you should be staying away from.

1. **Trans Fats & Hydrogenated:** These are damaged fats and are extremely detrimental to your health. These types of fats can be found in certain crackers, candies, baked goods, processed foods, and fried foods. Certain oils contain hydrogenated fats and should be avoided. These fats increase the bad kind of cholesterol, the LDL's while lowering the good kind of cholesterol, the HDL's. This can increase your risk of heart disease, and can lead to obesity.

2. **Saturated Fats:** Saturated fats in moderation are ok and especially if they are coming from healthy sources such as grass-fed beef or coconut oil, however they should be consumed less than the healthy monounsaturated fats such as olive oil or nuts and seeds. Extremely high amounts of saturated fats can lead to obesity, heart disease, and Type II Diabetes.

Smart Fat Guidelines:

So now that we know what fats we should be eating, and what fats we shouldn't be eating let's take a look at some smart fat guidelines to determine exactly how much of these healthy fats we should be including into our diets.

- With foods like dark chocolate and cheese keep these in moderation, and when consuming them consume two thumb's worth.

- If you are a yogurt or milk drinker, and are currently drinking fat free or low fat versions, swap out the low fat dairy and opt for the full fat. Keep the full fat to the recommended serving size per day.

- For oils, try to use 1 tablespoon. If you are using olive oil as a dressing, use 1 tablespoon of olive oil on your salad, and if you are cooking use 1 tablespoon of coconut oil to coat your frying pan.

- When consuming grass-fed beef stick to the 3 ounce serving suggestion.

- If you want to snack on heathy nuts and seeds, stick to 1 small handful.

- For a high fat food such as an avocado try to envision it in 4 servings, and consume ¼ of the avocado at a time. If you do not consume too many healthy fats throughout the day, then you can increase your intake to half of an avocado. It's hard to measure out a serving size of an avocado, so just do your best here.

It is recommended that you get roughly 20-30% of your daily calories from fat, and when you are consuming all healthy fat options in your diet this goal will be easy to tackle. Use the guidelines above to make measuring healthy fats easy.

Chapter 4:

A 30 day Meal Plan with Healthy Fats

Please note that recipes that are in bold have a corresponding recipe in the recipe section of this book

Week 1

	Day 1	Day 2	Day 3	Day 4	Day 5
Breakfast	Egg omelet made with coconut oil and spinach	**Chia Pudding**	**Overnight Oats**	Egg omelet made with coconut oil and spinach	**Chia Pudding**
Snack	Handful of walnuts	½ sliced avocado on toast	1 cup of full fat unsweetened yogurt	Celery sticks with 1 Tbsp. almond butter	Handful of walnuts
Lunch	**Tuna Salad**	Large salad with olive oil dressing, chicken breast, and pumpkin seeds	**Healthy Egg Salad**	Large salad with olive oil dressing, chicken breast, and pumpkin seeds	**Healthy Egg Salad**
Snack	1 cup of full fat unsweetened yogurt	Handful of almonds	Handful of walnuts	½ sliced avocado on toast	Celery sticks with 1 Tbsp. almond butter
Dinner	**Grass-fed burgers**	Wild caught salmon with 1 sweet potato and broccoli	Spaghetti squash with beans, ground turkey, and coconut oil	Chicken with whole wheat pasta and a **Creamy Walnut Sauce**	**Grass-fed burgers**

Week 2

	Day 6	Day 7	Day 8	Day 9	Day 10
Breakfast	**Breakfast Yogurt Parfait**	**Healthy French Toast**	**Overnight Oats**	Egg omelet made with coconut oil and spinach	**Hot Oats**
Snack	**5 Minute Guacamole** with carrot sticks	**Banana Walnut Shake**	1 cup of full fat unsweetened yogurt	Celery sticks with 1 Tbsp. almond butter	Handful of walnuts
Lunch	**Spicy Salmon Salad**	**Avocado Chickpea Sandwich**	**Healthy Egg Salad**	Large salad with olive oil dressing, chicken breast, and pumpkin seeds	**3 Bean Salad**
Snack	1 cup of full fat unsweetened yogurt	**Chia Pudding**	**Ants on a log**	½ sliced avocado on toast	Celery sticks with 1 Tbsp. almond butter
Dinner	**Grass-fed burgers**	**Chicken Stir Fry**	**Salmon Burgers**	**Stuffed Sweet Potato**	**Crock Pot Chicken with Gravy**

Week 3

	Day 11	Day 12	Day 13	Day 14	Day 15
Breakfast	Cinnamon Banana Pancakes	Hot Oats	Morning Rise Toast	Egg omelet made with coconut oil and spinach	Vegetarian Tofu Scramble
Snack	Chia Pudding	½ sliced avocado on toast	1 cup of full fat unsweetened yogurt	Banana Walnut Date Shake	Handful of walnuts
Lunch	Tuna Salad	Large salad with olive oil dressing, chicken breast, and pumpkin seeds	3 Bean Salad	Healthy Pasta Salad	Turkey Roll Up's
Snack	1 cup of full fat unsweetened yogurt	Yogurt Parfait	Chia Pudding	Trail Mix	Celery sticks with 1 Tbsp. almond butter
Dinner	Chicken Stir Fry	Wild caught salmon with 1 sweet potato and broccoli	Baby Back Ribs	Chicken with whole wheat pasta and a Creamy Walnut Sauce	Turkey Tacos

Week 4

	Day 16	Day 17	Day 18	Day 19	Day 20
Breakfast	**Breakfast Burrito**	**Morning Rise Toast**	**Overnight Oats**	Egg omelet made with coconut oil and spinach	**Overnight Oats**
Snack	**Trail Mix Apple**	½ sliced avocado on toast	1 cup of full fat unsweetened yogurt	**Trail Mix**	Handful of walnuts
Lunch	**Tuna Salad**	Large salad with olive oil dressing, chicken breast, and pumpkin seeds	**Turkey Roll Up's**	**Salmon Stir Fry**	**Roast Beef Italian Sandwich**
Snack	1 cup of full fat unsweetened yogurt	**Chia Pudding**	Handful of walnuts	½ sliced avocado on toast	**Ants on a log**
Dinner	**Stuffed Peppers**	**Grass Fed Burgers**	Spaghetti squash with beans, ground turkey, and coconut oil	**Salsa Chicken**	**Salmon Salad**

Week 5

	Day 21	Day 22	Day 23	Day 24	Day 25
Breakfast	Egg omelet made with coconut oil and spinach	**Hot Oats**	**Overnight Oats**	**Vegetarian Tofu Scramble**	**Breakfast Burrito**
Snack	**Spicy Avocado**	**Almond Butter Banana**	1 cup of full fat unsweetened yogurt	**Trail Mix Apple**	Handful of walnuts
Lunch	**Avocado Chickpea Sandwich**	Large salad with olive oil dressing, chicken breast, and pumpkin seeds	**Roast Beef Italian Sandwich**	**Healthy Steak Lunch**	**Healthy Egg Salad**
Snack	1 cup of full fat unsweetened yogurt	Handful of almonds	**Spicy Avocado**	½ sliced avocado on toast	**Almond Butter Banana**
Dinner	**Salmon Burgers**	**Stuffed Peppers**	**Stuffed Sweet Potato**	Chicken with whole wheat pasta and a **Creamy Walnut Sauce**	**Grass-fed burgers**

Week 6

	Day 26	Day 27	Day 28	Day 29	Day 30
Breakfast	**Breakfast Yogurt Parfait**	**Chia Pudding**	**Healthy Egg Omelet**	Egg omelet made with coconut oil and spinach	**Healthy Breakfast Smoothie**
Snack	**Trail Mix Apple**	½ sliced avocado on toast	1 cup of full fat unsweetened yogurt	Celery sticks with 1 Tbsp. almond butter	**Trail Mix**
Lunch	**Healthy Pasta Salad**	Large salad with olive oil dressing, chicken breast, and pumpkin seeds	**Turkey Roll Up's**	Large salad with olive oil dressing, chicken breast, and pumpkin seeds	**Healthy Egg Salad**
Snack	**Coconut Milk Smoothie**	Handful of almonds	Handful of walnuts	½ sliced avocado on toast	**Ants on a log**
Dinner	**Stuffed Sweet Potato**	Wild caught salmon with 1 sweet potato and broccoli	Spaghetti squash with beans, ground turkey, and coconut oil	Chicken Stir Fry	**Grass-fed burgers**

50 Delicious Healthy Fat Recipes

Breakfast

Overnight Oats

Servings: 2

Ingredients:

-1 cup of gluten free rolled oats

-1 cup of unsweetened almond milk

-1 Tbsp. of chia seeds

-1 tsp. pure vanilla extract

-1 Tbsp. of almond butter

Directions:

-Combine the oats with the rest of the ingredients minus the almond butter, and place in the fridge overnight.

-In the morning, serve with ½ Tbsp. of almond butter per serving.

Healthy Fat Breakfast Smoothie

Serves: 2

Ingredients:

-1 scoop of undenatured whey protein powder

-1/2 cup of almond milk plus ½ cup of coconut milk

-1 tsp. cocoa powder

-1 avocado

Directions:

-Core, the avocado and scoop out the avocado flesh, and place in the blender with the rest of the ingredients. Blend until smooth.

Healthy French toast

Serves: 1

Ingredients:

-2 slices of gluten free or whole wheat bread

-2 Tbsp. of coconut oil

-1 tsp. of cinnamon

Directions:

-Lather both sides of your bread with coconut oil, and sprinkle with the cinnamon.

-Heat a large skillet over medium heat, and cook both slices of bread until crispy.
Serve warm

Healthy Egg Omelet:

Serves: 1

Ingredients:

-2 whole, organic eggs

-2 Tbsp. of whole milk

-1/2 cup of fresh spinach

-1/4 cup of black beans

-1 Tbsp. of coconut oil.

Directions:

-Start by whisking the eggs, and milk together, and set aside.

-Heat a skillet over medium heat, and oil the pan with the coconut oil.

-Once the skillet is hot, pour the egg yolk mixture onto the pan, and let one side cook.

-While the one side is cooking, add the spinach, and beans.

-Flip one half of the omelet over, and let is cook for another 2-3 minutes.

Breakfast Yogurt Parfait:

Serves: 2

Ingredients:

-2 cups of full fat unsweetened yogurt

-1 cup of fresh berries

-2 Tbsp. of walnuts

-1 Tbsp. of honey

Directions:

-Simply layer your parfait, with the yogurt on the bottom and top with the fresh berries, walnuts and a drizzle of honey.

Hot Oats:

Serves: 1

Ingredients:

-3/4 cup of rolled oats

-1 cup of full fat coconut milk

-1 Tbsp. of slivered almonds

-1 tsp. of raisins

-1 tsp. of almond butter

Directions:

-Start by bringing the oats, and coconut milk to a boil, and continue to stir until cooked.

-Pour the hot oats into a serving bowl, and top with raisins, almonds, and almond butter.

Cinnamon Banana Pancakes

Serves: 3

Ingredients:

-1/2 of a banana

-1 egg

-1/2 cup coconut flour

-1 tsp. cinnamon

-1 tsp. nutmeg-

- 2 Tbsp. Peanut butter

-Coconut oil for cooking

Directions:

-Blend all ingredients minus the peanut butter. Cook 3 minutes each side in the coconut oil.

Morning Rise Toast

Serves: 1

Ingredients:

-2 Eggs

-2 slices of gluten free toast

-1/4 of an avocado

-Salt & pepper to taste

- Drizzle of olive oil

Directions:

-Start by whisking the eggs and cook them to your liking.

-Toast the bread, and smear with mashed avocado, top with egg and a drizzle of olive oil.

Vegetarian Tofu Scramble

Serves: 2

Ingredients:

-1/2 block of Tofu, extra firm

- ¼ cup of slices grape tomatoes-

-1/2 tsp. Cumin seeds

-2 Tbsp. of Tahini

-Coconut oil for cooking

-Salt and pepper to taste

Directions:

-Prepare the tofu by cutting into cubes, and sautéing with coconut oil, diced tomatoes, and cumin seeds.

When cooked, drizzle with tahini dressing.

Breakfast Burrito

Serves: 1

Ingredients:

-1 whole wheat tortilla- 8 inch whole wheat

-1 chicken breast

-1/4 cup black beans

-1/4 cup of diced tomatoes

-Onions

-2 Tbsp. of whole fat shredded cheese

-Pinch of salt

-Coconut oil for cooking

Directions:

Sauté the chicken breast in the coconut oil. Add in the onions, and sauté until translucent.

Assemble the burrito with the chicken, black beans, diced tomatoes, shredded cheese, and onions. Roll into a burrito.

Lunch

Healthy Egg Salad

Serves: 1

Ingredients:

-2 eggs, boiled and mashed

-1/2 of an avocado

-2 slices of gluten free or whole wheat bread

-2 pieces of sliced tomato

-Lettuce

Directions:

-Start by mashing your hard-boiled egg, and add in the avocado. Whisk until combined.

-Add the sliced tomato, and serve over a bed of lettuce.

Healthy Tuna Salad

Serves: 2

Ingredients:

-1 can of tuna

-2 Tbsp. of avocado based mayonnaise

-1 tsp. of Dijon mustard

-1 apple, peeled and diced

-1 stalk of celery, chopped

Directions:

-Drain the tuna from the can, and add to a mixing bowl. Mix the tuna, avocado mayonnaise, and mustard.

-Add in the chopped apple and celery

Spicy Salmon Salad

Serves: 2

Ingredients:

-1 can of wild caught salmon

-2 Tbsp. of avocado based mayonnaise

-1 tsp. of paprika

-1 pinch of salt and pepper

-Arugula

Directions:

-Mix the salmon with the mayonnaise, paprika, and salt and pepper.

-Serve over a bed of arugula

Avocado Chickpea Sandwich:

Serves: 1

Ingredients:

-1/2 of an avocado

-1/2 Tbsp. of Dijon mustard

-1/4 cup of chickpeas, mashed

-1/4 tsp. of cayenne pepper

-1 slice of gluten free or whole wheat bread

Directions:

-Start by mashing the chickpeas, and add the mustard, and cayenne pepper.

-Add chickpeas to 1 slice of bread, and top with ½ of a sliced avocado.

-Serve as an open faced sandwich.

3 Bean Salad

Serves: 4

Ingredients:

-1, 15 oz. can of black beans

-1/2 15 oz. can of chickpeas

-1 15 oz. can of kidney beans

-3 Tbsp. of extra virgin olive oil

-1 tsp. of cumin

-1 handful of fresh cilantro, chopped

-1/2 cup of diced cherry tomatoes, sliced

-1 pinch of salt and pepper

Directions:

-Rinse all of the beans, and place into a large mixing bowl, and add in all of the ingredients.

-Mix well, and let this sit in the refrigerator until cold.

Healthy Pasta Salad:

Serves: 6

Ingredients:

-1 box of gluten free or whole wheat fusilli pasta

-1/2 cup of diced grape tomatoes

-2 celery stalks, chopped

-1 handful of fresh basil, chopped

-1/4 cup of extra virgin olive oil

-1 Tbsp. of oregano

-1/2 cup crumbled feta cheese

Directions:

-Cook the pasta according to the box instructions, and drain.

-Rinse the pasta, and add to a large mixing bowl. Add in the remaining ingredients, except the feta cheese, and mix well.

-Top with feta cheese.

Turkey Roll Ups

Serves: 2

Ingredients:

-4 slices of organic turkey breast

-1/2 of an avocado

-2 slices of sliced organic cheese

-1/2 of a cucumber, sliced into 2 thin strips.

Directions:

-To make 2 servings, lay the turkey breast flat, and top it with mashed avocado, cheese, and the cucumber slice.

-Roll, and serve with tahini or Greek yogurt as a dip.

Salmon Stir Fry

Serves: 2

Ingredients:

-6 oz. of salmon

-1 Tbsp. of reduce sodium soy sauce

-1 tsp. sesame oil

-1 Tbsp. of coconut oil

-1 cup of broccoli florets

-1 cup of cauliflower florets

Directions:

-Start by steaming your vegetables for 5 minutes, or until tender, and set aside.

-Pre-heat your skillet over medium heat, and add coconut oil, and the salmon to the pan, and let cook to your liking.

-Allow the salmon to flake, and add in the sesame oil, soy sauce, and veggies.

Roast Beef Italian sandwich

Serves: 1

Ingredients:

-2 slices of organic, grass fed roast beef

-1 slice of fresh mozzarella cheese

-1 whole wheat ciabatta roll

-1 Tbsp. of balsamic vinegar

-1/2 of a sliced tomato

Directions:

-Assemble the sandwich by spreading the dressing on a ciabatta roll, and topping the roll with all of the ingredients.

-Place on a griddle to make a hot sandwich, or enjoy cold.

Healthy Steak Lunch

Serves: 1

Ingredients:

-3 oz. of steak, cut into thin strips.

-1 oz. of provolone cheese

-1 tsp. of worcestershire sauce

-6 asparagus spears

Directions:

-Cook your steak to your liking, and cut in into thin strips.

-While the steak is still hot, top with the provolone cheese, and worcestershire sauce.

-Serve with cooked asparagus.

Dinner:

Grass-Fed Burgers

Serves: 4

Ingredients:

-1 pound of grass fed beef

-1 tablespoon of reduced sodium soy sauce

-1 tablespoon of Italian seasoning

-1 pinch of salt and pepper

-2 avocados

-9 lettuce leaves

-1 tomato, sliced

Directions:

-Start by placing your grass fed beef into a mixing bowl, and mix in the soy sauce, Italian seasoning, salt and pepper. Form 4 patties.

-Cook burger patties to your liking, and top with ½ of an avocado each, sliced tomato, and lettuce leaves as the bun.

Salmon Burgers:

Serves: 6

Ingredients:

-¾ cup green onions

-1 handful of cilantro

-1 tsp. lemon juice

-1.5 cups chopped fresh spinach

-1 lb. fresh water salmon

-1 cup cooked quinoa

-1 tsp. Celtic or Himalayan sea salt

Directions:

-Place all ingredients into a food processor, and pulse until combined.

-Form into patties, and cook on a heated skillet for 3-4 minutes each side.

-Serve using lettuce as your "bun" with avocado, lettuce, and onion.

Chicken Stir Fry

Serves: 2

Ingredients:

-2 free range chicken breasts

- 1 cup of broccoli

-1 cup of snow peas

-2 carrots, serialized

-1 Tbsp. miso whisked with 1 tsp of Dijon mustard and 1 Tbsp. olive oil

-1 Tbsp. of coconut oil

Directions:

-Start by cutting the chicken into cubes, and place in a stir fry pan with the 1 Tbsp. of coconut oi. Cook until cooked through.

-While the chicken is cooking, steam the broccoli, and snow peas, and spiralizer the carrots with either a spiralizer, or a knife.

-Add the veggies to the stir fry pan which the chicken, and let this cook for 3 minutes.

-Whisk the miso, Dijon mustard, and 1 Tbsp. of olive oil together for the sauce.

-Add the sauce to the pan, and toss until combined.

Stuffed Sweet Potato

Serves: 2

Ingredients:

-2 large sweet potatoes

-3 Tbsp. of coconut oil

-1 cup of fresh spinach

-1 chicken breast, cut into cubes

-1 Tbsp. of reduced sodium soy sauce

Directions:

-Start by roasting the sweet potatoes in a 375 degree F oven for 40-45 minutes or until cooked through.

-While the sweet potatoes are cooking, cook the cubed chicken breast with 1 Tbsp. of coconut oil, and add the soy sauce once the chicken is cooked through.

-Add the fresh spinach to the pan, and cook until the spinach is wilted.

-After the sweet potatoes are finished cooked, slice down the middle, and dap with 1 Tbsp. of coconut oil each. Top with the spinach, and cubed chicken.

Crock Pot Chicken with Gravy

Serves: 6

Ingredients:

-4 pound organic kosher chicken

-2 tablespoons of ghee

-1 onion, chopped

-4 cloves of garlic

-1 tablespoon tomato paste

-1/2 cup chicken stock

- Pinch of salt and pepper

-1 Tablespoon of your favorite poultry seasoning

Directions:

-Start by heating a skillet over medium heat with the ghee. Add the onion, and garlic and sauté for 3 minutes.

-Next, add the tomato paste to the vegetables, season with salt and pepper, and add the chicken stock. Let this simmer for 5 minutes. Remove from heat, and let this sit in the fridge until you are ready to use it.

-Now add the entire chicken, breast side down to the crock pot, and season with your favorite poultry seasoning.

-Let this cook on low for 6 hours.

-Right before the chicken is done, take out the vegetables and stock, and blend with an immersion blender to create a gravy.

-Once the chicken is cooked, serve with the gravy and some steamed vegetables or sweet potato.

Baby Back Ribs

Serves: 2

Ingredients:

-1 rack of grass fed beef back ribs

-Seasoning rub of choice

-1 pinch of sea salt

-2 tablespoons of coconut aminos

Directions:

-Start by seasoning the ribs with the seasoning rub, salt, and coconut aminos, and placing them in a zip lock bag in the fridge for at least 3 hours.

-Broil the ribs for until charred on both sides, and cooked to your liking.

-Serve with fresh steamed vegetables, such as asparagus.

Turkey Tacos

Serves: 4

Ingredients:

-1 lb. lean ground organic turkey

-1 1.13oz Simply Organic Southwest Taco Seasoning packet

-¼ cup water

-8 lettuce leaves to use as "taco shells"

-1 cup sautéed kale

-1 avocado sliced

-1 Tbsp. olive oil

Directions:

-Start by sautéing your kale with the 1 Tbsp. olive oil.

-Cook the ground turkey until it is no longer pink.

-Add in the seasoning, the water and kale.

-Spoon tacos into shell, and top with the sliced avocado.

Stuffed Peppers

Severs: 4

Ingredients:

-2 red bell peppers

-2 orange or yellow bell peppers

-3 tbsp. extra-virgin olive oil

-1 red onion minced

-1 clove garlic minced

-1 lb. ground grass fed beef

-1 cup of cherry tomatoes

-1 tbsp. fresh oregano, minced

-1 tbsp. fresh cilantro, minced

-Sea salt and freshly ground black pepper to taste;

Directions:

-Preheat your oven to 350F.

-Cut 2 red bell peppers and 2 orange or yellow bell peppers in half. Remove the seeds and the white membrane. Wash the peppers thoroughly.

-Place the bell peppers on a cooking dish and apply 1 tbsp. of olive oil over the peppers.

-Cook the bell peppers for 20 minutes.

-While the peppers are cooking, pre-heat a skillet over medium heat, and sauté the garlic and onions for 2-3 minutes.

-Now, add the ground beef to the pan.

-When the meat is almost cooked through, add the cherry tomatoes fresh herbs and cook for another 5 minutes.

-Stuff all the pre-cooked bell peppers with the beef mixture.

-Cover the bell peppers with foil and place in the oven for 35 minutes.

Salmon Salad

Serves: 1

Ingredients:

-2 cups of mixed salad greens

-1/2 of an avocado

-½ ripe nectarine

-5 cherry tomatoes, sliced

-1 Tbsp. walnut halves

-3 oz. wild caught salmon, cooked

-1 Tbsp. of olive oil mixed with 1 Tbsp. of Dijon mustard for dressing

Directions:

-Preheat the oven to 400° degrees.

-Heat a pan over medium high heat until very hot.

-Add coconut oil. Once melted, place the salmon skin side down and cook until the salmon is no longer pink.

-While the salmon cooks assemble the lettuce with the remaining ingredients, chopping all of the ingredients into pieces.

-In a separate small bowl, combine the olive oil with the Dijon mustard for the dressing.

-Dress the salad with the dressing, and top with salmon.

Salsa Chicken

Serves: 6

Ingredients:

-2 cups organic salsa

-4 free range chicken breasts

-1 tbsp. chili power

-1 onion, chopped

-2 Tbsp. of coconut oil.

-1 cup of fresh spinach per serving.

Directions:

-Start by rinsing off the chicken, and season with the chili powder, and 1 cup of the salsa in a zip lock bag. Let the chicken marinate for 1 hour.

-After 1 hour, chop the onion, and sauté in a pan with coconut oil for 2-3 minutes, set aside.

-Next cook the chicken in another tablespoon of coconut oil over medium heat until cooked through.

-Add the remaining salsa, and onion and let this simmer for 5 minutes.

-Serve over a bed of spinach.

Snacks:

5 Minute Guacamole

Serves: 5

Ingredients:

-2 ripe avocados

-Juice of ½ of a lime

-½ red onion finely chopped

-Handful of fresh cilantro chopped

-Sea Salt & pepper to taste

Directions:

-Start by rinsing your cilantro, and then finely chopping the onion and cilantro, and place in a mixing bowl.

-Next cut, peel, and pit the avocados and add to the bowl.

-Next, juice the lime by cutting it in half, and squeezing the juice into the bowl. Add in a little salt and pepper and mash!

Banana Walnut Shake

Serves: 1

Ingredients:

-1 cup unsweetened almond milk

-½ cup ice

-½ frozen banana

-1 tsp. cinnamon

-1 Tbsp. crushed walnuts

-2 dates, pitted

-2 Tbsp. ground flax seeds

-1 scoop of whey protein powder

Directions:

-Place all ingredients into a high speed blender, and blend until smooth.

Ants of a Log

Serves: 2

Ingredients:

-6 celery sticks

-2 Tbsp. of raisins

-2 Tbsp. of almond butter

Directions:

-Wash the celery sticks, and smear 1 tsp. of almond butter on each celery stick. Top with 1 tsp. of raisins each.

Yogurt Parfait:

Serves: 2

Ingredients:

-2 cup of full fat yogurt

-1 cup of blueberries

-2 Tbsp. of chopped pecans or walnuts

-2 Tbsp. of honey

Directions:

-Scoop the yogurt into 2 serving bowls. Top the yogurt with ½ cup of blueberries each 1 Tbsp. of chopped nuts, and 1 Tbsp. of honey each.

-Serve chilled.

Chia Pudding:

Serves: 4

Ingredients:

-1 cup of unsweetened almond milk

-1/4 cup of chia seeds

-1 Tbsp. of cocoa powder

-1 tsp. of pure vanilla extract

Directions:

-Whisk the almond milk, and chia seed together in a large mixing bowl.

-Add in the cocoa powder, and vanilla, and stir until combined.

-Refrigerate for at least 2 hours before serving.

Homemade Trail Mix:

Serves: 6

Ingredients:

-1/2 cup of walnuts

-1/2 cup of pecans

-1/4 cup of cashews

-1 tsp of cinnamon

-1/2 cup of dark chocolate chips.

Directions:

-Place all ingredients into a large zip lock bag, and shake to combine.

Trail Mix Apples

Serves: 2

Ingredients:

-1 large apple sliced

-2 Tbsp. of honey

-2 Tbsp. of dark chocolate chips

-1 Tbsp. of chopped pecans

Directions:

-Wash, and slice your apple, and drizzle with the honey.

-Top with dark chocolate chips, and chopped pecans.

Spicy Avocado

Serves: 2

Ingredients:

-1 avocado, pitted and halved

-2 tsp. of hot sauce

-2 tsp. of olive oil

-1 tsp. of sea salt

-1/2 tsp of pepper

Directions:

-Top the avocado halves with olive oil, hot sauce, salt and pepper.

Almond Butter Bananas:

Serves: 2

Ingredients:

-1 large, ripe banana

-2 Tbsp. of almond butter

-1 tsp. of cinnamon

Directions:

-Peel the banana, and slice in half.

-Smear the almond butter on the banana, and sprinkle with cinnamon.

Coconut Milk Smoothie:

Serves: 1

Ingredients:

-1 cup of full fat coconut milk, canned

-1/2 cup of fresh or frozen strawberries

-1/2 frozen banana

-1 Tbsp. of honey

-8 ice cubes

Directions:

-Place all ingredients into a high speed blender, and blend until smooth.

Desserts:

Banana Ice Cream

Serves: 2

Ingredients:

-4 extra ripe frozen bananas

-1/4 cup of full fat coconut milk

-2 tsp. of cocoa powder

-Shredded coconut for topping

Directions:

-Place all ingredients into a high speed blender except for the shredded coconut, and pulse until the bananas form a soft serve ice cream consistency.

-Top with shredded coconut.

Coconut Ice Cream

Serves: 2

Ingredients:

-1 cup of full fat coconut milk ice cream

-2 tsp. of dark chocolate chips

-2 tsp. of chopped pecans

Directions:

-Scoop the coconut milk ice cream, and top with chocolate, and pecans.

Dark Chocolate Covered Almonds

Serves: 4

Ingredients:

-1 cup of dark chocolate

-2 cups of almonds

-Sea salt to taste

Directions:

-Melt the chocolate over a double broiler, or in the microwave.

-Stir in the almonds, until well coated.

-Place the almonds on a parchment lined baking sheet, and sprinkle with sea salt.

-Store in the fridge to set.

Dark Chocolate Coated Mangos:

Serves: 4

Ingredients:

-1/2 cup of melted coconut oil

-1/2 cup of raw cocoa powder

-2 Tbsp. of pure maple syrup

-1 tsp. of pure vanilla extract

-1 cup of dried mangos

Directions:

-Melt the coconut oil in a sauce pan over low heat, and stir in the cocoa powder, maple syrup, and vanilla.

-Stir in the dried mangos, and toss until coated.

-Place on a parchment lined baking sheet, and freeze for 20 minutes to let the chocolate set.

-Store any leftovers in the fridge.

Chocolate Covered Strawberries:

Serves: 4

Ingredients:

-1/2 cup of melted coconut oil

-1/2 cup of raw cocoa powder

-2 Tbsp. of honey

-2 cups of strawberries

-1/2 cup of shredded coconut

Directions:

-Melt the coconut oil in a sauce pan over medium heat, and add in the cocoa powder, and honey.

-Dip the strawberries into the chocolate mixture, to cover and then sprinkled with the shredded coconut.

-Place the chocolate covered strawberries on a large parchment covered baking sheet, and store in the fridge until ready to serve.

Sauces

Homemade Ketchup:

Serves: Makes 1.5 cups

Ingredients:

-1 can of tomato paste

- 2 Tbsp. of lemon juice

-1/4 tsp dry mustard

-1/3 cup water

-1 tsp. of ground allspice

Directions:

-Place all ingredients into a large bowl, and stir until combined.

-Store in the refrigerator

Mustard:

Serves: Makes ½ cup

Ingredients:

-1/2 cup mustard powder

-1/2 cup water

-1 Tbsp. of olive oil

-Sea salt to taste

Directions:

-Whisk all ingredients together, and store in the refrigerator.

Worcestershire sauce:

Serves: Makes ½ cup

Ingredients:

-1/2 cup apple cider vinegar

-2 tbsp. water

-2 tbsp. coconut aminos

-1/4 tsp mustard powder

-1/4 tsp onion powder

-1/4 tsp garlic powder

-1/8 tsp freshly ground black pepper

Directions:

Whisk all ingredients together in a mixing bowl until well combined.

Coconut Butter Spread

Serves: Makes ½ cup

Ingredients:

-1/2 cup of coconut butter

-1 Tbsp. of cinnamon

-1/2 tsp of sea salt

Directions:

-Stir the coconut butter, cinnamon and sea salt together.

-Store in an airtight glass container.

Creamy Walnut Sauce:

Serves:

Ingredients:

-4 Tbsp. of ghee

-1/2 cup of chopped, and soaked walnuts

-1 tsp. of sea salt

-1/2 cup of unsweetened almond milk

-1/4 cup of grated goat cheese

Directions:

-Soak the walnuts for at least 1 hour, or overnight.

-Place the soaked walnuts, and the remaining ingredients into a high speed blender, and blend until smooth.

Thank you so much for reading. I hope it added some value to your life.

Please take a moment and leave a review on Amazon.com

References

(1) https://www.nlm.nih.gov/medlineplus/ency/patientinstructions/000104.ht

m

(2) http://paleoleap.com/demolishing-fat-makes-fat-myth/

(3) http://drhyman.com/blog/2013/11/26/fat-make-fat/

(4) https://chriskresser.com/new-study-puts-final-nail-in-the-saturated-fat-

causes-heart-disease-coffin/

(5) http://www.fitnessmagazine.com/recipes/healthy-eating/tips/why-non-fat-

isnt-the-answer/

(6) http://authoritynutrition.com/10-super-healthy-high-fat-foods/

www.ingramcontent.com/pod-product-compliance
Lightning Source LLC
Chambersburg PA
CBHW071117280526
45787CB00003B/1079